RESISTANT
STARCH BIBLE

The Complete Resistant Starch
Diet And Cookbook Guide For Gut
Health, Gut Balance, Soluble
Fiber, Natural Antibiotics And A
Complete Well Being

Dr. Sheldon Mike

Table of Contents

CHAPTER 1

RESISTANT STARCH

Resistant starch is food that resists normal digestion within the intestine.

Lined with enzymes and digestive juices designed to interrupt foods up and absorb available nutrients, most foods are digested there. However, some foods are immune to the digestive power of the tiny intestine. These foods are resistant starches. Undigested within the intestine, these "super" starches actually find yourself feeding the great bacteria in your intestine.

To thrive, your intestine and therefore the bacteria within it must have proper fuel. Short-chain fatty acids especially one known as butyrate are the well-liked fuel for your internal system. To make butyrate, the massive intestine needs starch. But most starch is weakened within the intestine. Resistant starch which moves past the tiny intestine and into the massive intestine is vital for overall colon health because it's one among the sources for the eventual creation of butyrate. There are some simple ways to feature resistant starch to your diet.

FOOD SOURCES OF
RESISTANT STARCH

There are four different sources of resistant starch which are grouped consistent with their source: a. Type 1 is found within the fibrous cell walls of grains and seeds.

b. Type 2 is formed from raw starches; potatoes, green bananas and a few legumes.

c. Type 3 foods get their resistant starch from the cooking then cooling process. This includes sweet potatoes, rice, yams and a few whole grain breads.

d. Type 4 is man-made or chemically produced. This type is

usually employed by food manufacturers who add it to

EAT RIGHT

The best and most convenient way to get resistant starch within the diet is thru cooked then cooled potatoes and rice, unripe bananas, beans and legumes, sweet potatoes, yams and tubers. These are all essentially good carbs. Raw potato starch flour is additionally one among my favorites. It's available in many food stores and may be easily stirred into your morning glass of water or smoothie. if you're using raw potato starch that heat will destroy much of its benefit so cooking with it'll lessen its power. Some legumes like black beans, red lentils, and navy beans have adequate amounts of resistant starch, too. legume intake is strongly related to living an extended disease-free life.

CHAPTER 2

SIMPLE WAYS TO URGE MORE HEALTHY RESISTANT STARCH

* Add 1-2 tbsp of raw potato starch in your water or smoothies
* Add small amounts of potato starch to thicken puddings and non-dairy yogurts
* Mix potato starch to almond or coconut milk beverages
* Add slices of green banana to morning smoothies
* Incorporate unripe banana slices (they don't need to be completely green) into fruit salads
* Mix a minimum of 1 daily

serving of cooked legumes into salads, soups or have as a side

HEALTH BENEFITS OF RESISTANT STARCH

Resistant starch is simply too good to pass up. There are numerous health benefits for the whole body and it's just too easy to not increase the diet. The foremost important benefits includes:
a. Stay Full, Longer Similar to high-fiber or high-protein diets, resistant starch can keep you feeling full for extended . In light of the low-carb diet obsession, you'll are tempted to

chop out starchy foods completely, but healthy high-starch foods can actually assist you reduce, cut cravings and boost energy. Boost mineral absorption another exciting feature of resistant starch is how it improves absorption of minerals. Vital minerals like calcium and iron are commonly bound up in foods, making it hard for the body to soak up. Also, these are two minerals that are often deficient during a person's diet. When starch is fermented by gut bacteria, it creates an environment that permits minerals to be better absorbed.

c. The bathroom-related benefits resistant starch also can improve bowel function. Bowel irregularity, constipation or diarrhea can often be improved by adding resistant starch to the diet. Resistant starch isn't weakened by the tiny intestine, therefore when it passes to the massive intestine it is food for all of our good gut bacteria.

These bacteria are the key to a healthy digestion. They actively prevent diarrhea, cramping and help create soft bulky stools. This makes resistant starch the right solution for anyone who has had to line up shop within the bathroom due to dense and hard bowel movements.

d. Cancer Prevention Possibly the foremost important reason to feature resistant starch to your diet is for possible protection against a deadly enemy:

* colorectal cancer. This is where much of the resistant-starch research has focused on the consequences of resistant starches to enhance bowel health, promote good bacteria and ultimately prevent bowel cancers from forming.

CHAPTER 3

UNDERSTANDING THE WORD- STARCH

Starch may be a chain of glucose molecules, a sequence of sugar molecules. Once you eat starch, you've got enzymes in your body that cut those chains. Imagine having a true chain linked together. We've enzymes that break the starch chain apart then your body can use these individual links, which are sugars. These starches are often found in foods like potatoes and rice and grains. Most starch is digested, but alittle portion is resistant and that is what we call resistant starch.

SORTS OF RESISTANT STARCH

* Type 1

Resistant starch type one is found in cell walls. It's physically inaccessible and it's found in minimally processed whole grains, seeds, and beans. They are present in beans also. Just confirm to cook beans properly because they contain lectins, which may irritate the gut. While not most are vulnerable to this gut irritation from lectins, it's something that we all got to concentrate to, especially if we've autoimmune diseases or other problems with the gut. Once you refine grains an excessive amount of , that's getting to cause you to possess more digestible starch and it is also getting to cause your blood glucose to rise. Stick with minimally processed foods and cook them properly.

* Type 2

Resistant starch type two isn't digestible to sugar because it's a crystalline structure. It's found in raw potatoes and green bananas for instance. Generally, fruits aren't meant to be eaten when they are not ripe. Think about this natural cycle: fruits are naturally meant to be eaten when they're ripe because by then, the seeds would be able to spread to grow another tree, so trees create chemicals within the fruits that cause you to not want to eat them.

LITTLE FACTS YOU SHOULD KNOW

Nature prevents you from eating fruits that haven't reached its optimum state for consumption. With green bananas, however, there's probably an exception to the present rule. It's most probable that given the utilization of green bananas in traditional cultures and therefore the amount of resistant starch in them, the advantages outweigh any negatives.

* Raw potatoes have a toxic chemical in them and we're not certain if the supplements out there actually reduce this chemical and you have to avoid raw potato starch.

* Type 3

Resistant starch type three is retrograded starch, my favorite type. It's formed once you take starch found in polished rice and sweet potatoes; you cook them, and then refrigerate them overnight. This cooking and refrigerating process creates resistant starch.

As a result, calories are reduced slightly and it's getting to blunt the blood glucose rise when you're eating these foods. It allows you to enjoy sweet potatoes and rice during a while every so often every now and then and again from time to time occasionally sometimes infrequently once in a while in a healthier way when it involves blood glucose .

* Type 4

Resistant starch type four may be a modified starch that's made by the food industry. Again, we would like to stay to minimally processed foods, with many greens and properly cooked beans and seeds. If you've got these in your diet, you are going to urge enough variety that the gut bacteria are getting to prey on, which can create those chemicals which will be beneficial to your body. While getting resistant starch from an entire host of various plants, you're also producing chemicals that benefit your health. It's just amazing to me that each single day within the medical literature, we're finding that it isn't necessarily the foods that we're eating that contain the top product that's causing such a lot benefit; it's actually what the great bacteria within the gut are forming or creating in response to eating all of those fibers from different sorts of plants that make a difference. The lignans in flaxseeds for instance aren't processed into short-chain fatty acids, but instead form compounds which will have positive hormonal effects within the body. Gut bacteria that churn out an entire host of chemicals that affect everything from hormones to blood glucose to your mood. Your job is to form sure they   get   the   proper   food.

CHAPTER 4

WHAT YOU NEED TO UNDERSTAND

What makes resistant starch different from fiber the reality is, some people consider resistant starch to be a kind of fiber. But Miracle Noodles, it might be classified as a non-starch polysaccharide.

This means that although it isn't made from a sequence of glucose molecules like resistant starch, it actually is formed from a sequence, but not just glucose. it is also immune to digestion within the sense that it's also forming and allowing the beneficial bacteria to make short-chain fatty acids, which goes to make this healthy lining of the gut and make gut barrier. It'll even have these anti-inflammatory effects.

CONCLUSION

The best way to urge resistant starch is to use type 3, the retrograded starch or to include green bananas into your diet. The retrograded starch is where you're taking a starch, an honest one like sweet potatoes or polished rice and you cook it, and then refrigerate it overnight.

THE END

Made in the USA
Monee, IL
06 May 2024

58033306R00015